Spaghetti Squash Recipes

About the Author

Laura Sommers is **The Recipe Lady!**

She is the #1 Best Selling Author of over 80 recipe books.

She is a loving wife and mother who lives on a small farm in Baltimore County, Maryland and has a passion for all things domestic especially when it comes to saving money. She has a profitable eBay business and is a couponing addict, avid blogger and YouTuber.

Follow her tips and tricks to learn how to make delicious meals on a budget, save money or to learn the latest life hack!

Visit her blog for even more great recipes and to learn which books are FREE for download each week:

http://the-recipe-lady.blogspot.com/

Visit her Amazon Author Page to see her latest books:

amazon.com/author/laurasommers

Laura Sommers is also an Extreme Couponer and Penny Hauler! If you would like to find out how to get things for **FREE** with coupons or how to get things for only a **PENNY**, then visit her couponing blog **Penny Items and Freebies**

http://penny-items-and-freebies.blogspot.com/

© Copyright 2017. Laura Sommers.
All rights reserved.
No part of this book may be reproduced in any form or by any electronic or mechanical means without written permission of the author. All text, illustrations and design are the exclusive property of
Laura Sommers

About the Author ii

Introduction 1

Baked Spaghetti Squash Lasagna 2

Italian Spaghetti Squash 3

Paleo Spaghetti Squash 4

Spicy Spaghetti Squash 5

Spaghetti Squash Saute 6

Southwestern Spaghetti Squash 7

Paprika Chicken Spaghetti Squash 8

Spaghetti Squash and Cucumber Salad 9

Sicilian Spaghetti Squash Salad 10

Spaghetti Squash Primavera 11

Feta Spaghetti Squash Casserole 12

Avocado and Egg Spaghetti Squash Boats 13

Eggs And Spaghetti Squash 14

Eggs In A Spaghetti Squash Nests 15

Spaghetti Squash Frittata 16

Spaghetti Squash Noodle Salad with Peanut Sauce 17

Spaghetti Squash Hash Browns 18

Alfredo Spaghetti Squash 19

Mushroom Parmesan Spaghetti Squash 20

Creamy Tomato Spaghetti Squash 21

Spaghetti Squash Chow Mein 22

Spaghetti squash with chèvre 23

Garlic Spinach Spaghetti Squash 24

- Spaghetti Squash Pad Thai 25
- Chicken & Spaghetti Squash 27
- Spaghetti Squash Shrimp Scampi 28
- Mushroom Lentil Spaghetti Squash Casserole 29
- Spaghetti Squash Greek Salad 31
- Spinach, Kale And Spaghetti Squash Fritters 32
- Spaghetti Squash Tacos 34
- Thai Red Curry Chicken Spaghetti Squash Bowls 35
- Chorizo Ragu Stuffed Spaghetti Squash 36
- Spaghetti Squash Burrito Bowls 37
- Pesto Shrimp Spaghetti Squash 38
- Pesto Chicken Spaghetti Squash 39
- Spaghetti Squash Kugel 40
- Spaghetti Squash Patties 41
- Cinnamon Spaghetti Squash Cake 42
- Spaghetti Squash Indian Dessert (Kheer) 43
- Spaghetti Squash "Bread" Pudding 44
- Spaghetti Squash Rice Pudding 45
- Spaghetti Squash Pie 46
- Spaghetti Squash Mock Coconut Pie 47
- Spaghetti Squash Bread 48
- Beef Spaghetti Squash Bake 49
- Scalloped Spaghetti Squash 50
- Spinach and Spaghetti Squash Quiche 51
- Spaghetti Squash with Asparagus 52
- About the Author 53
- Other books by Laura Sommers 54

Introduction

Spaghetti squash is a is a large yellow squash, so named because the inner flesh separates in to spaghetti-like strands when scraped out with a fork after being cooked. If you enjoy spaghetti but are trying to limit your pasta intake due to calories or carbs, then you already have two reasons to eat spaghetti squash as a replacement. A cup of cooked spaghetti squash has only 42 calories while a cup of cooked pasta has over 200 calories. It is high in fiber and low in calories which help aid in weight loss.

Here are some other reasons to eat spaghetti squash:

It is rich in antioxidants. This versatile squash contains vitamin A and vitamin C, which can help prevent free radical damage to cells. Spaghetti squash is also rich in the B vitamins riboflavin, niacin, and thiamin, which promote optimal cellular function.

Other antioxidants found in spaghetti squash variety are beta-carotene, lutein, and zeaxanthin, which are all linked to healthy vision and optimal eye health. Beta-carotene can also prevent atherosclerosis by lowering the cholesterol levels. It is also beneficial for people with insulin resistance.

It is ideal for pregnant women in that it contains folate which helps prevent birth defects.

Spaghetti squash promotes cardiovascular health since it is high in potassium and helps lower high blood pressure. It contains omega-3 and omega-6 fatty acids to help prevent heart diseases, inflammation, arthritis and different types of cancers. It is good for prostate health, and it can also be used for treating benign prostate enlargement.

Spaghetti squash has very little taste itself, so it takes on the flavors of whatever you cook with it. In this recipe book, you will find tons of great recipes for spaghetti squash so that you can enjoy all the benefits of this great Super Food!

Baked Spaghetti Squash Lasagna

Ingredients:

1 spaghetti squash, halved lengthwise and seeded
1 onion, chopped
2 tbsps. minced garlic
2 (14 oz.) cans stewed tomatoes
1 tbsp. dried basil
1 cube vegetable bouillon black pepper to taste
1 (15 oz.) can black olives, chopped
1 cup shredded mozzarella cheese
1 cup shredded Parmesan cheese

Directions:

1. Preheat oven to 325 degrees F (165 degrees C).
2. Spray a baking sheet with a thin layer of cooking spray.
3. Place squash halves cut side down on the baking sheet.
4. Bake squash 35 minutes in the preheated oven, or until a knife can be easily inserted. Remove from oven, and cool.
5. Meanwhile, spray a non-stick saucepan with cooking spray.
6. Over medium heat, saute the onion and garlic until golden brown.
7. Stir in tomatoes, basil, bouillon cube, and black pepper.
8. Cook for about 15 minutes, or until you have a medium thick sauce.
9. Remove squash strands with a fork, reserving the shells. Layer each half with a spoonful of the sauce, a layer of spaghetti squash strands, olives, and mozzarella cheese.
10. Repeat layers until shells are full, or until all of the ingredients are used.
11. Top with Parmesan cheese.
12. Bake for 20 minutes in the preheated oven, or until Parmesan cheese melts.

Italian Spaghetti Squash

Ingredients:

1/2 cup water
1 spaghetti squash, halved and seeded
2 tbsps. butter
1 tbsp. olive oil
1 onion, diced
1 clove garlic, minced
1 (14.5 oz.) can diced tomatoes with onion, celery, and green pepper
2 tsps. dried basil
1 tsp. salt
1 tsp. ground black pepper
1/4 cup shredded Parmesan cheese, plus more for topping

Directions:

1. Preheat oven to 350 degrees F (175 degrees C).
2. Pour water in baking dish and place halved squash cut-sides down in the dish.
3. Bake squash in preheated oven until a fork pierces the skin very easily, about 45 minutes. Let squash cook while preparing remainder of recipe.
4. Melt butter with olive oil in a large skillet over medium-high heat.
5. Saute onion in hot butter until softened, about 5 minutes.
6. Add garlic and continue to saute until fragrant, about 1 minute more. Pour diced tomatoes over the onion mixture; season with basil.
7. Place a cover on the skillet, reduce heat to medium-low, and cook at a simmer until the tomatoes are soft, about 30 minutes; season with salt and pepper.
8. Once squash is cool enough to handle, use a fork to strip flesh from the skin in strands.
9. Stir squash and Parmesan cheese into tomato mixture.
10. Replace cover on skillet and cook until squash is heated through, 5 to 10 minutes more.
11. Sprinkle additional Parmesan cheese over the dish to serve.

Paleo Spaghetti Squash

Ingredients:

2 spaghetti squash, halved and seeded
1/4 cup olive oil, or as needed
Salt and ground black pepper to taste
2 sausages 1 (15 oz.) can diced tomatoes
1 tomato, diced 2 cloves garlic, minced
4 oz. baby spinach leaves

Directions:

1. Preheat oven to 375 degrees F (190 degrees C). Line a baking sheet with aluminum foil.
2. Season squash halves with olive oil, salt, and black pepper.
3. Place squash, cut-side down, on prepared baking sheet.
4. Bake in the preheated oven until tender, about 1 hour.
5. Cool squash for 10 minutes; scrape flesh out of squash with a fork.
6. Cook and stir sausages in a skillet over medium heat until no longer pink in the center, 7 to 10 minutes.
7. An instant-read thermometer inserted into the center should read 160 degrees F (70 degrees C).
8. Stir spaghetti squash, canned tomatoes, diced tomato, and garlic into skillet with sausages; cook and stir until warmed-through, 2 to 4 minutes.
9. Add spinach; cook and stir until spinach wilts, 2 to 4 minutes. Season with salt and black pepper.

Spicy Spaghetti Squash

Ingredients:

1 spaghetti squash, halved and seeded
2 tbsps. olive oil, divided
2 tbsps. chopped fresh parsley
1 tbsp. red pepper flakes
Salt and ground black pepper to taste

Directions:

1. Preheat oven to 350 degrees F (175 degrees C).
2. Coat the inside of squash with about 1 tbsp. olive oil.
3. Place squash, cut-side down, on a baking sheet.
4. Bake in the preheated oven until squash is tender, about 30 minutes. Cool squash for 10 minutes.
5. Shred the inside of squash with a fork and transfer to a bowl.
6. Add remaining olive oil, parsley, red pepper flakes, salt, and pepper to shredded squash.
7. Toss to coat.

Spaghetti Squash Saute

Ingredients:

Cooking spray
1 spaghetti squash, halved and seeded
1/4 cup butter or margarine
1 small onion, chopped
2 cloves garlic, finely chopped
Salt and pepper to taste

Directions:

1. Preheat an oven to 350 degrees F (175 degrees C).
2. Coat a baking sheet with cooking spray, and place squash halves cut-side down on the sheet.
3. Bake until squash is tender but still crunchy, about 40 minutes.
4. Set aside to cool.
5. Once cool enough to handle, shred squash flesh from rind using a fork. Set aside.
6. Melt butter in a skillet over medium heat. Cook onion and garlic in butter until soft.
7. Add squash to the skillet, and cook until hot.
8. Season with salt and pepper.

Southwestern Spaghetti Squash

Ingredients:

1 spaghetti squash, halved and seeded
1 tbsp. olive oil
Olive Oil
1 (15 oz.) can black beans, rinsed and drained
2 tomatoes, chopped
1 green bell pepper, chopped
1 clove garlic, minced
1 tbsp. olive oil
1 tbsp. red wine vinegar
1/4 cup chopped fresh cilantro
Salt and pepper to taste

Directions:

1. Preheat an oven to 425 degrees F (220 degrees C).
2. Place squash halves in a shallow baking pan with about 1 inch of water.
3. Bake squash in the preheated oven until soft, about 1 hour.
4. Scrape flesh of squash from the rind using a fork and place in a large serving bowl.
5. Heat 1 tbsp. olive oil in a large skillet over medium heat. Cook and stir the black beans, tomatoes, bell pepper, and garlic in the hot oil until the vegetables are soft and the liquid has reduced, about 10 minutes; pour into the bowl with the squash; toss to combine.
6. Add 1 tbsp. olive oil, the vinegar, and cilantro and toss again. Season with salt and pepper to serve.

Paprika Chicken Spaghetti Squash

Ingredients:

1 (3 pound) spaghetti squash
2 tbsps. olive oil
1 onion, thinly sliced
2 cloves garlic, minced
1 green bell pepper, diced
2 tbsps. paprika
1 tsp. salt 1 tsp. caraway seeds
Ground black pepper to taste
3 skinless, boneless chicken breast halves
1 (14.5 oz.) can whole peeled tomatoes, drained
1/2 cup sour cream

Directions:

1. Preheat oven to 350 degrees F (175 degrees C).
2. Using a skewer or fork, pierce squash in several places.
3. Place whole squash on a baking sheet; roast for 45 minutes. Turn squash over and roast for an additional 10 minutes. Set aside to cool.
4. Heat olive oil in a large skillet over medium-high heat.
5. Cook and stir onion, garlic, green bell pepper, paprika, salt, caraway seeds and ground black pepper in the hot oil until onion is soft and translucent, about 5 minutes.
6. Remove from skillet and set aside, leaving olive oil in pan.
7. Reduce heat to medium and cook chicken breasts in the same skillet until browned, the juices run clear, and meat is no longer pink inside, turning once, about 10 minutes per side.
8. Remove chicken breasts and slice on the diagonal.
9. Return chicken and onion mixture to the pan; stir in tomatoes. Bring chicken mixture to a simmer.
10. Slice squash in half and scoop out seeds with a spoon.
11. Using a fork, scrape spaghetti-like strands of squash from the peels.
12. Combine squash with chicken and vegetables, increase heat, and bring to a boil.
13. Reduce heat to low and simmer to combine flavors, about 10 minutes.
14. Stir in sour cream if desired.

Spaghetti Squash and Cucumber Salad

Ingredients:

1 spaghetti squash, halved and seeded
8 oz. cherry tomatoes, halved
6 oz. pitted kalamata olives, halved
2 English cucumbers, peeled, seeded, and sliced
1 small red onion, sliced thin
1 clove garlic, minced
1/4 cup lemon juice
1 tbsp. lemon zest
1/4 cup olive oil, or more if needed
1 tbsp. garlic
Salt ground black pepper to taste

Directions:

1. Preheat an oven to 350 degrees F (175 degrees C).
2. Place the squash halves into a large baking dish with the cut-sides facing down.
3. Bake in the preheated oven until you can easily cut into the skin side with a knife, about 30 minutes.
4. Remove from oven and set aside to cool.
5. Toss the cooled spaghetti squash, the tomatoes, olives, cucumbers, red onion, and garlic together in a large bowl until evenly mixed.
6. Stir the lemon juice and lemon zest together in a small bowl.
7. Slowly pour the olive oil into the lemon juice mixture while whisking vigorously.
8. Season with garlic salt and pepper; drizzle over the spaghetti squash mixture and toss to coat.
9. Refrigerate at least 2 hours before serving.

Sicilian Spaghetti Squash Salad

Ingredients:

1 spaghetti squash water as needed
1 1/2 cups crumbled Macedonian feta cheese   cup slivered roasted red bell peppers
1 cup slivered sun-dried tomatoes 3/4 cup chopped Kalamata olives 2/3 cup chopped fresh basil
1/2 cup chopped fresh parsley
1/3 white onion, chopped 1 jalapeno chile pepper, diced 3 tbsps. Greek salad dressing 3 tbsps. balsamic vinegar 2 tbsps. white wine vinegar 2 tbsps. extra-virgin olive oil
1 tbsp. chopped fresh thyme 1 tbsp. minced garlic 1 1/2 tsps. ground black pepper 1 tsp. salt

Directions:

1. Preheat oven to 350 degrees F (175 degrees C).
2. Slice spaghetti squash lengthwise and scoop out seeds. Place cut-side down in a baking dish; add 1/2 inch water.
3. Bake in the preheated oven until fork tender, about 35 minutes. Cool squash until easily handled.
4. Shred spaghetti squash from rind using a fork; cool to room temperature.
5. Combine feta cheese, red bell peppers, sun-dried tomatoes, Kalamata olives, basil, parsley, white onion, and jalapeno pepper together in a large bowl. Stir in Greek salad dressing, balsamic vinegar, white wine vinegar, olive oil, thyme, garlic, ground black pepper, and salt. Add spaghetti squash; toss to combine.

Spaghetti Squash Primavera

Ingredients:

1 spaghetti squash 2 tbsps. extra-virgin olive oil
1 onion, choppe
1 large clove garlic, minced 1 large zucchini, cut into bite-size pieces
1 green bell pepper, chopped 1 tbsp. dried Italian herb seasoning fresh ground black pepper, to taste   1/2 cups chopped tomato 3/4 cup crumbled feta cheese

Directions:

1. Pierce the shell of the spaghetti squash with a fork and place in a microwave-safe dish; cook in microwave on High for 12 minutes. Set aside to cook until cool enough to handle. Slice in half lengthwise; remove the seeds. Use a fork to pull the flesh of the squash away from the shell and place into a large bowl; fluff with the fork to separate the strands as much as possible.
2. Heat the olive oil in a large skillet over medium heat. Cook and stir the onion in the hot oil until just tender, about 3 minutes. Add the garlic and continue cooking and stirring another 3 minutes. Stir the zucchini and green bell pepper into the mixture; season with the Italian herb seasoning and black pepper. Pour the tomatoes into the skillet. Continue cooking just until the tomatoes are warmed, 3 to 5 minutes. Add the squash to the skillet and toss until evenly mixed. Sprinkle with the feta cheese and toss again to serve.

Feta Spaghetti Squash Casserole

Ingredients:

1 spaghetti squash, halved and seeded salt and ground black pepper to taste
3 Roma tomatoes, diced 1 small onion, diced
1 cup crumbled feta cheese 2 cups spinach, or more to taste   1/2 cups spaghetti sauce
1 cup shaved Parmesan cheese

Directions:

1. Preheat oven to 350 degrees F (175 degrees C). Place squash face down in a baking pan; pour in water to 1/2 inch.
2. Bake in the preheated oven until interior can be easily pierced with a fork, about 1 hour. Cool until easily handled, about 15 minutes.
3. Scrape squash flesh into spaghetti strands with a spoon; place into a bowl. Season with salt and pepper.
4. Spread squash, tomatoes, onion, feta cheese, spinach, and spaghetti sauce in 3 even layers in a casserole dish. Top with Parmesan cheese.
5. Bake in the preheated oven until Parmesan cheese is melted and bubbly, 30 minutes to 1 hour.

Avocado and Egg Spaghetti Squash Boats

Ingredients:

1 small spaghetti squash
4 tbsp salsa, divided
1 avocado, chopped & divided Coupons
2 large eggs
4 tbsp low sodium ketchup, divided

Directions:

1. Preheat oven to 400 F degrees F. Cut spaghetti squash in half lengthwise and scoop the seeds out. Place cut side down on a baking sheet lined with parchment paper and bake for 30 minutes. Remove from the oven and let cool until safe to the touch, about 15 minutes.
2. Increase oven temperature to 425 degrees F. Using a fork, separate spaghetti squash into strands leaving them inside the shells. Add 2 tbsp of salsa to each half and mix gently with a fork. Top with 1/2 avocado and break 1 egg on top of each shell. If you like runny egg yolk, do not make a well in the middle of the squash and break the egg on top. For a fully baked egg, sink it more into squash. Bake for 20 - 22 minutes or until the egg whites appear to be set. Serve hot drizzled with ketchup.

Eggs And Spaghetti Squash

Ingredients:

1 C spaghetti squash
1 tsp ghee
2-3 hard boiled eggs
Fresh herbs
Salt + Pepper

Directions:

1. Cook spaghetti squash by preferred method. I poke several holes in the squash with a sharp knife. Microwave for 5 minutes, and let it sit for 3 minutes. Rotate and flip over the spaghetti squash in the microwave and cook for 5 more minutes. Let squash sit for about 10 minutes, or until cool enough to handle.
2. Cut spaghetti squash in half. Remove and discard seeds. Scrape out squash with a fork. Let squash sit in a colander to allow water to drain.
3. Put 1 C of spaghetti squash in a bowl. Store remaining squash in the refridgerator for 1-2 weeks.
4. Top spaghettis squash with eggs and ghee. Warm in microwave to melt ghee, and stir gently to combine squash with eggs.
5. Season with fresh herbs (pictured with rosemary), salt and pepper to taste.

Eggs In A Spaghetti Squash Nests

Ingredients:

1¾ cups cooked spaghetti squash (see how to cook spaghetti squash)
1 tbsp. olive oil
1 medium yellow onion, minced
8 eggs plus 1 egg white
1 tsp. garlic powder
1 tsp. kosher salt
⅛ tsp. ground black pepper
2 tbsp. chickpea flour (can also use coconut flour or another gluten-free flour)
⅓ cup Parmesan, grated

Directions:

1. Preheat the oven to 425.
2. Place the cooked spaghetti squash in a large mixing bowl and set aside.
3. In a fry pan, heat the olive oil over medium-high heat. Once hot, add the onion and cook until tender, about 4-6 minutes.
4. Add the onion to the bowl with spaghetti noodles, along with the egg white, garlic powder, salt, pepper, flour, and cheese, and mix well.
5. Scoop a little less than ¼ cup of the noodle mixture into each muffin tin. Using your fingers or a spoon, press the squash noodles down and around the sides of the muffin cup. This will create your nest.
6. Place the nests into the oven and bake for 16-20 minutes, or until the top edges become golden and crispy.
7. Reduce the heat to 375 and remove the muffin tin from the oven.
8. Crack 1 egg into each tin, taking care not to overflow the nest.
9. Return to the oven and bake for an additional 10 minutes, or until the egg whites are fully cooked and no longer transparent. (For fully cooked-through eggs, cook 2-5 minutes longer).

Spaghetti Squash Frittata

Ingredients:

1 small spaghetti squash (2 cups shredded)
3 eggs
1 c kale, chopped
1/2 c mushrooms, sliced
1/4 c white onion, diced
1/2 tsp oregano
sea salt and fresh ground black pepper to taste

Directions:

1. To prepare the spaghetti squash, preheat oven to 350F.
2. Wash and slice the squash in half and place cut sides down onto a baking sheet.
3. Roast about 25-30 minutes or until fork tender.
4. Shred with a fork into a medium sized bowl and set aside.
5. Lightly spray or grease a small frying pan and add in chopped mushrooms and onion and sauté over medium heat for about 3-4 minutes. When onions are translucent and fragrant remove from pan and set aside.
6. Crack the eggs into the bowl with the squash and add the spices. Mix until combined.
7. Mix in the kale, mushrooms and onion and then pour the mixture into the same frying pan, cover and cook over medium heat for about 8 minutes or until eggs are cooked through.
8. Remove frittata from heat, slice and plate to serve.

Spaghetti Squash Noodle Salad with Peanut Sauce

Ingredients:

1/2 small spaghetti squash, halved and seeded
1/3 cup peanut butter
2 tbsps. tamari
1/2 tsp. agave syrup
1/4 tsp. sea salt
1/4 tsp. minced fresh ginger
1/4 tsp. minced garlic
1/2 lime, juiced
1 dash sriracha hot sauce (optional)
1 cup shredded cabbage
1 cup chopped broccoli
1 small cucumber, cut into matchstick-size pieces
1 carrot, shredded
2 scallions, minced
1 sprig fresh mint, thinly sliced
1/4 cup roasted, salted peanuts

Directions:

1. Preheat oven to 400 degrees F (200 degrees C).
2. Place squash, cut-side down, on a baking sheet.
3. Bake in the preheated oven until squash is tender, about 30 minutes. Cool until easily handled.
4. Combine peanut butter, tamari, agave syrup, sea salt, ginger, and garlic in a microwave-safe bowl.
5. Heat in microwave until sauce is smooth, about 1 minute.
6. Stir lime juice and sriracha into sauce.
7. Shred squash into a large bowl using a fork or your fingers.
8. Add cabbage, broccoli, cucumber, carrot, scallions, and mint.
9. Drizzle peanut sauce over mixture and toss to coat.
10. Top salad with peanuts.

Spaghetti Squash Hash Browns

Ingredients:

2 cups spaghetti squash, cooked and shredded
1 tbsp. oil

Directions:

1. Heat the oil in a large non-stick skillet over medium heat
2. Press the water out of the squash with paper towels
3. Form little patties by pressing the squash firmly between your palms
4. Place the patties gently on the warmed skillet and let cook for 5-7 minutes per side.
5. Transfer to paper towels to drain, then serve warm

Alfredo Spaghetti Squash

Ingredients:

1 (3 lb.) spaghetti squash
1 head of cauliflower, cut into small florets
4 tbsp. + 3 tbsp. chicken stock, divided
1/2 cup minced white onion
1 1/2 tbsp.. minced garlic
2 tsp olive oil
1 cup coconut cream
1 tsp salt
1/2 tsp. pepper
1/4 tsp. nutmeg
3 tbsp. lemon juice

Directions:

1. Preheat the oven to 400 degrees F.
2. Boil some water in a large pot and put the cauliflower florets into it.
3. Let the cauliflower cook for 11 minutes, strain, and set aside.
4. While the cauliflower is cooking, cover a cookie sheet in aluminum foil.
5. Cut the spaghetti squash in half and remove the mushy core with a spoon. Then cover the surface with some olive oil and evenly "paint it on" with a silicone basting brush.
6. Lay the squash face down on the aluminum paper.
7. Cook the spaghetti squash for 35 minutes and then remove it from the oven and let cool.
8. Add cauliflower into a food processor with 4 tbsps. chicken stock.
9. Puree the cauliflower in the food processor and then set the mashed cauliflower aside.
10. Put 2 tsp of olive oil in a large pan over medium-high heat.
11. Put the minced onion and garlic into the pan and mix into the olive oil. Cook for 3 minutes, while mixing often.
12. Reduce the heat to medium, and add the coconut cream, pureed cauliflower, 3 tbsps. of lemon juice, and 3 Tbs of chicken stock to the pan and mix. Add the salt, pepper, and nutmeg, mix and then let the mixture cook for 10-15 minutes, until you have the desired consistency.
13. Using two forks, "rake" against the inside of the squash until the insides looked like "spaghetti".
14. Put all of the spaghetti squash into a large bowl.
15. Top with alfredo and serve.

Mushroom Parmesan Spaghetti Squash

Ingredients:

1 small spaghetti squash
2 tbsps. extra virgin olive oil
2 cups button mushrooms, chopped bite size
2 garlic cloves, finely chopped
1 tbsp. fresh thyme
¼ cup parmesan cheese, grated
1 handful flat leaf parsley, finely chopped
salt and pepper to taste

Directions:

1. Preheat oven to 380 degrees F
2. In a deep skillet (or large pan), add olive oil, garlic and thyme.
3. Cook for 2 minutes over high heat and add mushrooms. Cook until mushrooms are golden brown (about 7-8 minutes). Turn off the heat and set aside.
4. Put the spaghetti squash on a baking tray and pierce a the skin a few time using a knife. Bake for about an hour, until squash can be pierced with a knife. Alternatively, you can microwave the spaghetti squash. Instructions are at the bottom.
5. Take squash out of the oven and let cool to room temperature. Cut in half and get rid of the seeds. Use a fork to scrape the squash into strings.
6. Add squash to the skillet (or pan), turn the heat to high and quickly fry with mushrooms. Sprinkle parmesan while sauteing for a minute.
7. Turn the heat off, top with parsley and season with salt and pepper. Serve.
8. Microwaving spaghetti squash: Place spaghetti squash on a microwave safe plate or other microwave safe container. Place the cut side down (skin facing up). Microwave on high for 10 minutes.
9. Take the spaghetti squash out of the microwave and shred with a fork.

Creamy Tomato Spaghetti Squash

Ingredients:

Spaghetti squash Ingredients:

1 medium spaghetti squash
2 tsp extra virgin olive oil
2 tsp minced garlic
Salt
Ground pepper

Tomato Sauce Ingredients:

½ cup raw cashews, soaked
1-15 oz. can diced fire roasted tomatoes
¼ cup basil leaves, chopped
2 tbsps. water
½ tsp salt
Red pepper flakes, optional

Directions:

1. Place cashews in a bowl and cover with water.
2. Allow them to soak for at least 2 hours or overnight.
3. Preheat oven to 375 degrees F.
4. Slice spaghetti squash in half. Scoop out seeds and stringy flesh with a spoon.
5. Rub a tsp. of olive oil over each half (inside, not outside).
6. Rub with garlic and sprinkle with salt and pepper.
7. Place face down on a baking sheet and bake for 35 minutes.
8. Meanwhile, place the sauce ingredients in a blender and blend until completely smooth and creamy.
9. Set aside.
10. Use a fork to shred the spaghetti squash into strands.
11. Heat a pan over medium heat.
12. Place squash in a pan and cover with sauce.
13. Toss to combine until warmed through.
14. Top with fresh basil and red pepper flakes prior to serving.

Spaghetti Squash Chow Mein

Ingredients:

1 large spaghetti squash
1/4 cup coconut aminos (or tamari if not paleo)
3 cloves garlic, minced
1 tbsp. coconut sugar
2 tsps. freshly grated ginger
1/4 tsp. pepper
2 tbsps. olive oil
1 onion, diced
3 stalks celery, sliced diagonally
2 cups coleslaw mix

Directions:

1. Cut a spaghetti squash in half length wise and scoop out seeds.
2. Lay skin side up in a 13 x 9 pyrex and pour 1/2 inch of water in the bottom of the pan. Bake at 400 degrees for 30-40 minutes, until flesh is very tender.
3. Once done, scoop out flesh with a fork so it breaks apart into strings, set aside.
4. In a small bowl, whisk together coconut aminos, garlic, coconut sugar, ginger and white pepper; set aside.
5. Heat olive oil in a large skillet over medium high heat.
6. Add onion and celery, and cook, stirring often, until tender, about 3-4 minutes.
7. Stir in cabbage until heated through, about 1 minute.
8. Stir in spaghetti squash and sauce mixture until well combined, about 2 minutes.

Spaghetti squash with chèvre

Ingredients:

1 large spaghetti Squash, cut in half lengthwise seeds scooped out
1 small shallot
3 tbsps. extra-virgin olive oil
2 tbsps. lemon juice
2 tsps. honey
2 tsps. fresh chopped thyme
½ tsp. salt
½ tsp. freshly ground pepper
¼ cup sliced toasted almonds
2 oz. fresh chèvre (goat cheese), crumbled

Directions:

1. Place spaghetti squash in a 9 by 11 baking dish, cut-side down.
2. Pour one cup water in the pan. Cover with a layer of parchment or wax paper.
3. Cover with plastic wrap.
4. Microwave until the spaghetti squash pulls apart into tender threads when tested with a fork, 16 to 20 minutes.
5. Meanwhile, puree shallot, oil, lemon juice, honey, thyme, salt and pepper in a mini prep, with an immersion blender or in a blender.
6. When squash is tender, carefully remove the cover, and transfer the squash to a cutting board with tongs. Scrape spaghetti squash out of the shell with the forks.
7. Mound on a platter or plates.
8. Drizzle all over with dressing, top with almonds and chevre.

Garlic Spinach Spaghetti Squash

Ingredients:

1 spaghetti squash
2 tbsps. olive oil
3 cloves garlic, minced
2 pints grape tomatoes
4 cups of spinach
toasted pine nuts, optional
Parmesan cheese, optional
Himalayan sea salt, to taste

Directions:

1. Preheat oven to 400 degrees F.
2. Cut squash in half lengthwise and discard seeds.
3. Place on a parchment-lined baking sheet, cut-side down, and roast for 30–45 minutes.
4. On another parchment-lined baking sheet, spread tomatoes and drizzle with 1 tbsp. olive oil. Roast for 15–20 minutes.
5. When squash is finished cooking, allow to cool then, using a fork, scrape the squash to get long spaghetti-like strands
6. In a large sauté pan, heat olive oil over medium heat, add garlic, and stir until fragrant.
7. Turn down heat to low and add tomatoes, spinach, and squash and continue to sauté 3–5 minutes. Season with Himalayan sea salt to taste.
8. Serve with pine nuts and Parmesan cheese on top.

Spaghetti Squash Pad Thai

Ingredients:

1 large spaghetti squash
Olive oil
Kosher salt
Fresh ground black pepper
3 carrots
½ red pepper
4 cloves garlic
5 green onions
2 eggs
½ cup chopped fresh cilantro
3 tbsps. sweet chili sauce
3 tbsps. soy sauce
1 lime
Sriracha (optional)
2 tbsps. peanut oil
1 and ½ cup bean sprouts, divided
½ cup roasted salted peanuts, chopped

Directions:

1. Preheat oven to 400 degrees F.
2. Using a large, sharp knife, cut the spaghetti squash in half.
3. Scrape out the seeds using a spoon and sprinkle the cut sides with olive oil.
4. Season with kosher salt and freshly ground black pepper.
5. Place the squash cut side down on a baking sheet and roast until tender and easily pierced with a knife, about 45 minutes. When the squash is done, use a fork to scrape out the flesh of each half into "noodles".
6. Place the noodles in a colander or sieve and drain for 10 minutes to remove the extra moisture.
7. Meanwhile, peel and shred 3 carrots. Thinly slice ½ red pepper.
8. Mince 4 cloves garlic. Thinly slice 4 green onions. In a small bowl, beat together 2 eggs.
9. Separately, thinly slice 1 green onion and chop ½ cup of fresh cilantro.
10. In another small bowl, mix together 3 tbsps. sweet chili sauce, 3 tbsps. soy sauce, juice of ½ lime, and if desired, a few dashes of Sriracha.
11. When the squash is ready, in a large skillet heat 2 tbsps. peanut oil over medium high heat.

12. Add the garlic and green onions cook until fragrant, about 45 seconds. Pour in the eggs and scramble until almost cooked.
13. Add the red pepper, carrots, 1 cup bean sprouts, and squash noodles. Add 3 pinches kosher salt and toss together.
14. Pour on the sauce and stir to combine. Cook about 2 minutes, until the vegetables are heated through but still crisp.
15. Garnish with crushed peanuts, fresh bean sprouts, cilantro, and green onion.

Chicken & Spaghetti Squash

Ingredients:

1 medium spaghetti squash (4 lbs.)
1 can (14-1/2 oz.) diced tomatoes, undrained
2 tbsps. prepared pesto
1/2 tsp. garlic powder
1/2 tsp. Italian seasoning
1/4 cup dry bread crumbs
1/4 cup shredded Parmesan cheese
1 pound boneless skinless chicken breasts, cut into 1/2-inch cubes
1 tbsp. plus 1 tsp. olive oil, divided
1/2 pound sliced fresh mushrooms
1 medium onion, chopped
1 garlic clove, minced
1/2 cup chicken broth
1/3 cup shredded cheddar cheese

Directions:

1. Cut squash in half lengthwise; discard seeds.
2. Place squash cut side down on a microwave-safe plate. Microwave, uncovered, on high for 14-16 minutes or until tender.
3. Meanwhile, in a blender, combine the tomatoes, pesto, garlic powder and Italian seasoning. Cover and process until blended; set aside. In a small bowl, combine bread crumbs and Parmesan cheese; set aside.
4. In a large skillet, cook chicken in 1 tbsp. oil until no longer pink.
5. remove and keep warm. In the same skillet, saute mushrooms and onion in remaining oil until tender.
6. Add garlic; cook 1 minute longer.
7. Stir in the broth, chicken and reserved tomato mixture.
8. Bring to a boil.
9. Reduce heat; simmer, uncovered, for 5 minutes.
10. When squash is cool enough to handle, use a fork to separate strands.
11. In a large ovenproof skillet, layer half of the squash, chicken mixture and reserved crumb mixture.
12. Repeat layers.
13. Bake, uncovered, at 350 degrees F for 15 minutes or until heated through. Sprinkle with cheddar cheese. Broil 3-4 in. from the heat for 5-6 minutes or until cheese is melted and golden brown.

Spaghetti Squash Shrimp Scampi

Ingredients:

Ingredients:

2 spaghetti squashes
8 tbsps. butter, divided
1½ pounds peeled and deveined large fresh shrimp
2 large shallots, minced
3 cloves garlic, minced
1 cup dry white wine
½ cup chicken broth
½ cup heavy whipping cream
2 tbsps. capers
1 tsp. Creole seasoning
¼ tsp. crushed red pepper
¼ cup chopped fresh parsley

Directions:

1. Preheat oven to 375 degrees F.
2. Line a baking sheet with aluminum foil.
3. Prick squashes all over with a fork. Place on prepared baking sheet, and roast until tender, about 1 hour and 20 to 30 minutes.
4. Let cool 15 minutes, then slice in half lengthwise. Use a fork to shred squash and place flesh in a large bowl, discarding seeds and skins.
5. In a large skillet, melt 1 tbsp. butter over medium-high heat.
6. Add shrimp and cook, turning occasionally, until pink and firm, about 5 minutes. Remove shrimp and set aside.
7. Melt 1 tbsp. butter in skillet over medium-high heat. Add shallots and garlic; cook, stirring occasionally, 6 minutes.
8. Add wine and broth, increase heat to high, and reduce liquid by two-thirds.
9. Reduce heat to medium-low.
10. Stir in remaining 6 tbsps. butter, cream, capers, Creole seasoning, and red pepper.
11. Cook until butter has melted and sauce is smooth, about 3 minutes.
12. Stir in squash, shrimp, and parsley. Serve immediately.

Mushroom Lentil Spaghetti Squash Casserole

Ingredients:

3 lb. spaghetti squash sliced in half lengthwise with seeds removed
1/2 cup dried red or green lentils
1 cup vegetable broth
1 c. white onion diced
3 cloves garlic minced
8 oz. button mushrooms stems removed & sliced
1/2 oz. block tofu
1/2 c. unsweetened plain non-dairy milk
1 1/2 tbsp. liquid aminos or tamari
1/2 tsp. dried sage
1/4 tsp. dried thyme
3 c. kale chopped with ribs removed
Salt and pepper to taste
1 tbsp. nutritional yeast
1 tbsp. instant oats

Directions:

1. Preheat your oven to 375 degrees F.
2. Place the two squash halves, cutside-down, into a large baking dish.
3. Fill the baking dish with a 1/4" of water and poke holes in the rinds of the squash, using a fork.
4. Once the oven is to temperature, bake for 30-40 minutes, or until the rind is soft.
5. While the squash is baking, bring the vegetable broth to a boil in a small pot over high heat.
6. Add the lentils in and return to a boil, then reduce heat to a simmer. Cover and cook for 20 minutes or until soft.
7. In a large, non-stick saute pan, heat the onion and garlic over medium, until the onions begin to clear.
8. Add the mushrooms to the pan and saute until soft, about 3-4 minutes.
9. Blend the tofu and non-dairy milk together until very smooth. Add it to the saute pan along with the liquid aminos, sage, and thyme.
10. Stir together and bring to a simmer. Adjust the heat to low-medium and fold in the chopped kale. Once the lentils are done cooking, stir them into the pan, as well.
11. Turn off the stove and take the pan off of the heated burner.

12. When the squash is cooked, take it out of the oven and adjust oven temperature to 350 degrees F.
13. Wait 10 minutes before scraping the squash from the rind with a fork into a colander to let the excess liquid drip out.
14. Add the squash to the saute pan and fold the mixture together.
15. Season with salt and pepper to taste and place it in an 8" square casserole dish.
16. Sprinkle the nutritional yeast and instant oats over the top and bake for 15-20 minutes.

Spaghetti Squash Greek Salad

Ingredients:

For the Salad
1 small to medium sized spaghetti squash, roasted and cooled.
1 cucumber, peeled, deseeded, and diced
1/2 cup cherry tomatoes, cut in half
1/2 cup roasted red pepper, diced
2 tbsps. shallot, minced
1/4 cup kalamata olives, diced
3 tbsps. feta cheese
For the Dressing
1 tsp. extra virgin olive oil
2 tbsps. red wine vinegar
2 tsps. freshly squeezed lemon juice
1 tsp. honey, more to taste
1/4 tsp. garlic powder
1/2 tsp. kosher salt
Freshly ground black pepper to taste

Directions:

1. Preheat oven to 400 degrees.
2. Line a baking sheet with foil and spray it with cooking spray.
3. Split the spaghetti squash in half and scrape out the seeds.
4. Spray the flesh of the squash with cooking spray and sprinkle with salt.
5. Lay the squash cut side down on the baking sheet and bake for 40 minutes.
6. Remove from the oven and let the squash cool to room temperature before scraping out the flesh with a fork.
7. In the meantime dice up the cucumber, roasted red pepper, kalamata olives, shallot, and cherry tomatoes.
8. In a small bowl whisk together all of the dressing ingredients.
9. Once the squash has cooled scrape out the flesh into a large bowl.
10. Add in the vegetables and dressing and toss together.
11. Top the salad with feta.

Spinach, Kale And Spaghetti Squash Fritters

Ingredients:

2-pounds spaghetti squash, cooked and shredded
1 tbsp. butter
1 tbsp. extra virgin olive oil
1 bell pepper, diced
1 pinch of salt
2 garlic cloves, minced
2 cups fresh baby spinach, packed
2 cups torn kale leaves, packed
Salt and fresh ground pepper, to taste
1/4 cup grated parmesan cheese
1/4 cup all-purpose flour
1/4 cup panko bread crumbs
1 egg, lightly beaten
1/8 tsp. seasoned salt
1/4 tsp. dried oregano
2 tbsps. chopped fresh parsley
Olive oil cooking spray
Plain nonfat yogurt for serving, optional

Directions:

1. Preheat oven to 425 degrees F.
2. Line 2 baking sheets with foil and grease with olive oil cooking spray.
3. Set aside.
4. In the meantime, prepare the greens mixture.
5. Heat butter and olive oil in a large nonstick skillet; add diced peppers and salt and continue to cook 3 to 4 minutes, or until peppers begin to soften.
6. Add garlic and cook for 1 minute or until fragrant.
7. Stir in spinach and kale; season with salt and pepper, and cook for 2 to 3 minutes, or until wilted.
8. Remove from heat and transfer to a mixing bowl; let stand a few minutes to cool.
9. Add spaghetti squash strands to the spinach mixture, as well as the parmesan cheese, flour, panko bread crumbs, egg, seasoned salt, oregano and parsley; mix until thoroughly combined.
10. Place in the fridge for several minutes, or until slightly cooled.

11. Remove from fridge and spoon mixture into 2 to 3-inch rounds on previously prepared baking sheets.
12. Lightly spray tops of rounds with olive oil cooking spray.
13. Bake for 10 minutes; flip the fritters over and continue to cook for 8 to 10 more minutes, or until browned on top.
14. Continue to do the same with the second baking sheet.
15. Remove from oven and transfer fritters to a serving plate.
16. Serve and enjoy!

Spaghetti Squash Tacos

Ingredients:

1 medium spaghetti squash
1 tbsp. freshly squeezed lemon juice
1/2 tbsp. chili powder
1/2 tsp ground cumin
1/2 tsp ground coriander
1/2 tsp sea salt
16 (6") corn tortillas
1 can organic black beans, rinsed and drained
1 cup Greek yogurt
1 cup cherry tomatoes, finely diced
1 avocado, chopped
Chopped cilantro
Salsa

Directions:

1. Preheat oven to 375 degrees and spray pan with coconut oil cooking spray.
2. Cut the squash in half lengthwise, scoop out the seeds and roast the halves facedown on baking pan for 35-40 minutes or until flesh is soft.
3. Once the squash is cooked, remove and allow to cool 5 minutes, then scrap the flesh with a fork to loosen and separate the strands. Add strands of flesh to bowl and discard skins.
4. In a separate bowl, combine chili powder, cumin, coriander, and salt, whisk in lemon juice and pour over squash strands. Gently toss to mix seasonings throughout, taste and adjust seasonings accordingly.
5. Heat a dry skillet over medium heat and warm tortillas one at a time until slightly blistered on each side, about 30-45 seconds per side.
6. To assemble the tacos, transfer warmed tortillas to platter and add spoonful of black beans, scoop of seasoned squash, dollop of Greek yogurt, finely chopped tomatoes and avocados, then sprinkling with chopped cilantro.
7. Add salsa, hot sauce or any other desired garnishes and serve.

Thai Red Curry Chicken Spaghetti Squash Bowls

Ingredients:

1 spaghetti squash, halved and seeded
1 chicken breast, thinly sliced
1 red bell pepper, seeded and thinly sliced
2 cup green snap peas or thinly sliced bamboo shoots
1 onion, sliced in ½" strips
½ cup fresh basil, chopped
1 green onion, chopped
1 cup chicken broth
2 tsp cornstarch
1 can light coconut milk
1 tbsp. red curry paste, more or less if desired
1 tbsp. olive oil
Lime Juice for garnish
Salt and Pepper to taste

Directions:

1. Place the spaghetti squash in a microwave safe baking dish, cut side down, and add 3 tbsps. water to the dish.
2. Cover dish with plastic wrap, venting slightly, and microwave to steam for 13 minutes, or until fork tender. It may take longer depending on your microwave, so check and continue cooking if necessary.
3. While the squash is cooking, in a large non-stick skillet over medium-high heat, heat up olive oil. Salt and pepper the thinly sliced chicken breast. Once oil is shiny, place into the pan and cook quickly allowing the chicken to brown on all sides. Once finished, set aside on plate.
4. In the same pan, add in vegetables (except basil) and cook until softened over medium-high heat, stir frequently. When softened but still crisp, set aside on same plate as the chicken.
5. While pan is hot, add in curry paste, and whisk in chicken broth, coconut milk, and corn starch. When the mixture begins to simmer and thicken, add in chicken and vegetables and basil. Reduce the heat and allow to simmer until the squash is done in the microwave.
6. When squash is done, invert the squash bowls, fill with red chicken curry and devour.

Chorizo Ragu Stuffed Spaghetti Squash

Ingredients:

2 small spaghetti squash, halved and seeds removed
2/3 lb. chorizo sausage, casings removed
2 garlic cloves, minced
1-1/2 tsp ground cumin
1/2 tsp smoked paprika
1 jalapeno, seeds and veins removed and minced
1/2 small yellow onion, diced
1 red bell pepper, diced
2 Roma tomatoes, diced
1 (14 oz.) can black beans, drained and rinsed
2-4 cups of spinach, stems removed and chopped
1/4 cup fresh cilantro, chopped
Juice from 1/2 lime
Salt and pepper, to taste
Garnish/serving ideas

Directions:

1. Preheat oven to 400 degrees F.
2. Lightly drizzle olive oil over squash and season with salt and pepper. Place squash cut side down onto a baking sheet lined with foil and bake for 30-35 minutes or until tender.
3. Set aside for serving.
4. While squash cooks, place a medium skillet over medium heat and add chorizo and onion.
5. Saute until cooked through and no longer pink and lightly browned.
6. Add garlic, cumin, paprika and jalapeno and cook until fragrant, about 30 seconds to one minute.
7. Add bell pepper, tomato and beans and cook for 3-4 minutes. Toss in spinach and cook another minute or two until wilted.
8. Add cilantro the the skillet along with fresh squeezed lime juice. Season to taste with salt and pepper.
9. Spoon ragu into cooked spaghetti squash. Sprinkle with grated cheese and/or additional cilantro if desired and enjoy!

Spaghetti Squash Burrito Bowls

Ingredients:

2 medium sized spaghetti squash
1 tbsp. high heat oil
1 (14.5 oz.) can black beans, drained and rinsed
1 (16 oz.) jar of salsa
2 tbsps. olive oil
1 large bell pepper or two small, cored and sliced
1 large red onion, sliced
2 cups corn kernels
1 cup fresh cilantro, finely chopped
2 jalapenos, cored and sliced
6 green onions, sliced
1 tsp. cumin
Salt and pepper
1 cup shredded cheddar cheese

Directions:

1. Preheat the oven to 375 degrees F and line a cookie sheet with foil.
2. Cut each squash in half lengthwise and then use a spoon to scrap out the seeds and the darker yellow strands that the seeds are attached to.
3. Rub a little bit of high heat oil on the inner edges of the squash and then place each half face down on the baking sheet.
4. Roast in the oven for 30-45 minutes, depending on the size.
5. Warm 1 tbsp. oil in a large pan over medium heat.
6. Sauté the red onion for a few minutes and then add the peppers and jalapeno.
7. Sprinkle with salt & pepper and cumin and cook to desired softness.
8. Remove from oven,
9. Turn the oven to broil and then transfer the squash to a surface where you can scrape the inside and begin stuffing.
10. Scrape about 3/4 of the inside out onto a dish and then layer the filling inside (black beans and corn, peppers and onion, salsa and cilantro).
11. Top with the spaghetti squash and press down then add another layer of filling.
12. Sprinkle green onion on top and then finish with shredded cheese.
13. Broil in the oven for about 5 minutes so that the cheese is bubble and golden brown.

Pesto Shrimp Spaghetti Squash

Ingredients:

1 medium-large spaghetti squash
1/3 cup pesto (homemade or store bought)
1 cup frozen peas, thawed
1/2 lb. frozen shrimp, thawed
salt and pepper, to taste
1 tsp. olive oil, if needed
1/4 cup Parmesan cheese

Directions:

1. Preheat oven to 375 degrees F.
2. Line a baking sheet with aluminum foil and spray with cooking spray.
3. Cut each squash in half lengthwise.
4. Remove the seeds and inner pulp of the squash.
5. Place spaghetti squash cut side down on prepared baking sheet.
6. Bake for 45 minutes at 375 degrees F.
7. Thaw the peas and shrimp by running under cold water for several minutes.
8. Add shrimp and cook for 1-2 minutes on each side.
9. Add peas to the saute pan to warm through.
10. Turn off heat and add the pesto, stirring to combine.
11. Season with salt and pepper, to taste.
12. Once the spaghetti squash has cooked and is cool enough to handle, take a fork and pull strands from the outer skin of each squash half.
13. Top the spaghetti squash with the warm pesto-pea-shrimp mixture.
14. Top with Parmesan cheese.

Pesto Chicken Spaghetti Squash

Ingredients:

2 spaghetti squash
2 heaping cups cooked shredded chicken (from 2 chicken breasts or a rotisserie chicken)
1/2 cup pesto (homemade or store bought)
1 pint cherry tomatoes, halved
Parmesan cheese for topping
Chopped fresh parsley for topping
Chopped basil leaves for topping

Directions:

1. Preheat the oven to 375 degrees F.
2. Cut each squash in half lengthwise.
3. Remove the seeds and inner pulp of the squash,
4. Place spaghetti squash cut side down on a baking sheet.
5. Bake spaghetti squash for 35-45 minutes, until squash is tender.
6. Combine shredded chicken and pesto and stir well.
7. Remove the spaghetti squash from the oven. Use a fork to scrape the inside of the squash lengthwise to make strands that look like spaghetti. Just be careful - it's hot!
8. Add the pesto chicken to the top of each spaghetti squash boat. Return to the oven and cook for 5-7 minutes, until warmed through.
9. Remove, top with the halved cherry tomatoes and serve, either directly in the spaghetti squash boat or transferred to a bowl.

Spaghetti Squash Kugel

Ingredients:

4 cups cooked spaghetti squash
3 eggs
1/2 cup (85gm) coconut sugar
2 tsps. cinnamon
2 apples, peeled, cored, and thinly sliced
1/3 cup raisins

Directions:

1. Preheat oven to 375°F. Spray an 8x8" baking dish with cooking spray, or lightly grease with melted coconut oil.
2. In a large bowl, whisk together eggs, coconut sugar, and cinnamon. Add spaghetti squash and toss to coat. Mix in apples and raisins. Pour the mixture evenly into the prepared baking dish.
3. Bake for 45 minutes or until golden and set. Cool before slicing.

Spaghetti Squash Patties

Ingredients:

1 cup Baked Spaghetti Squash (click for recipe), cooked and drained of excess water
2 whole Eggs, beaten
Salt and Pepper, to taste
Butter or oil for frying

Directions:

1. Squeeze and drain the spaghetti squash in paper towel.
2. Mix together squash and beaten eggs.
3. Heat ghee, coconut oil, or butter in frying pan.
4. Spoon mixture into frying pan.
5. Cook until golden brown and flip.
6. Cook until browned on second side.

Cinnamon Spaghetti Squash Cake

Ingredients:

1 small spaghetti squash
1 cup spelt flour
2 tsps. baking powder
1/4 tsp. baking soda
1 tsp. cinnamon
1 tsp. ginger
1/2 tsp. ground allspice
1/2 cup maple syrup
1/4 cup coconut oil
2 tbsps. flax meal
6 tbsps. water

Directions:

1. Preheat oven to 375 directions F.
2. Using a fork, pierce the spaghetti squash a few times around the outside and then microwave for three minutes. Cut the ends off the squash and cut the squash in half. Fill a large glass baking pan with water and place the two squash halves, flesh-side down into the pan.
3. Cover with foil and bake for about 25 minutes. The squash will be done when it is easy to piece the outside with a fork. Let cool a few minutes, remove seeds. Using a fork, scrape the inside of the squash to remove the strands of squash. Measure out 2 cups of squash and set aside.
4. Reduce oven heat to 350°F.
5. Spray an 8×8-inch baking pan with cooking spray and set aside.
6. In a small bowl combine the flax meal and water.
7. In a medium bowl stir the spelt, baking powder, baking soda, cinnamon, ginger, and allspice together.
8. In another small bowl whisk the maple syrup and coconut oil together. Add in the flax egg. Stir.
9. Mix the wet ingredients with the dry. Fold in the squash.
10. Baking about 25-28 minutes or until a toothpick comes out clean. Let cool before serving.

Spaghetti Squash Indian Dessert (Kheer)

Ingredients:

2 cans Organic Coconut Milk (full fat)
3 cups of spaghetti squash strands
1 tbsp. Ghee
1 tsp. freshly ground cardamom seeds, remove pod, just use seeds
3 tbsps. honey
Golden raisins
Sliced almonds

Directions:

1. Prepare spaghetti squash using the oven method (below) to achieve "noodles".
2. Heat ghee in pan and stir-fry the dry spaghetti squash strands.
3. Then, stir-fry nuts and raisins.
4. In another saucepan, add coconut milk and bring it to a boil.
5. Reduce the heat slightly, add honey, ground cardamom and stir.
6. After about 10-15 minutes, once the milk has thickened a bit, add the ghee-coated spaghetti strands.
7. Stir for a few more minutes, garnish with ghee-coated nuts and raisins and then serve.
8. To prepare squash using the oven method:
9. Preheat oven to 375.
10. Cut the squash in half, scoop out the seeds, and brush on some ghee to the cut sides.
11. Place squash cut side down in a baking dish.
12. Bake for 45 minutes or until you can easily pierce the skin with a knife

Spaghetti Squash "Bread" Pudding

Ingredients:

6 cups cooked spaghetti squash
3/4 cup milk
3 large eggs
3/4 cup Splenda
1 tbsp. pumpkin pie spice
1 tsp. vanilla extract

Directions:

1. Cook spaghetti squash.
2. Cut in half and remove seeds.
3. Remove pulp from shell.
4. Place in large mixing bowl.
5. Beat eggs until lemon colored and add to squash in bowl.
6. Add remaining ingredients and mix well.
7. Spray 8 X 8 baking dish. Turn mixture into dish.
8. Bake about 30 minutes at 350 degrees F, until browned and center is set.
- Add dried fruit, such as raisins if desired.

Spaghetti Squash Rice Pudding

Ingredients:

1½ lb. spaghetti squash
6 cups milk
1 cup rice
½ Sugar
2 tbsp Butter
¼ tsp salt
Cinnamon for garnish (optional)

Directions:

1. Chop the squash into 2 inch chunks and place them into a pot.
2. Remove the skins and seeds before adding them to the pot.
3. Add the milk to the chopped squash and let it sit over medium heat until it comes to a slight boil.
4. Add the sugar and salt to the pot and stir it in well.
5. Let it cook for another 15 minutes.
6. Once the squash has softened, add the rice and keep over medium heat until the rice is cooked. About 20-25 minutes.
7. Once the rice is cooked, add in the butter and enjoy.

Spaghetti Squash Pie

Ingredients:

2 cup cooked spaghetti squash
2 eggs
1/2 cup sugar
2 tsp. lemon extract
1/4 cup lemon juice
1/2 cup corn meal
1 baked pie shell

Directions:

1. Boil whole spaghetti squash about 30-45 minutes.
2. When cooked and cooled, cut lengthwise in half. Scoop out seeds.
3. With fork, shred out inner squash. It will look like spaghetti.
4. Beat 2 eggs, sugar, lemon extract, and juice together.
5. Fold in 2 cups of spaghetti squash. Add cornmeal and mix together.
6. Pour into baked pie shell and bake at 350 degrees for 30 minutes.
7. Test for doneness.

Spaghetti Squash Mock Coconut Pie

Ingredients:

1/2 cup sugar
8 packs Sweet & Low
4 eggs
1/4 cup diet butter
1/2 cup plain all-purpose flour
2 cup skim milk
1/4 tsp. salt
1/2 tsp. baking powder
1 tsp. vanilla flavoring
1 tsp. coconut flavoring
4 cups cooked, shredded spaghetti squash
Omit salt and baking powder if using self-rising flour.

Directions:

1. Cut squash in half - lengthwise - and remove seeds. Put cut side down in a pot with 2 inches of water. Cover and boil 20 minutes.
2. Microwave: Place squash cut sides down in a dish with 1/4 cup water. Cover with clear wrap and cook 7-8 minutes.
3. Run fork over inside of cooked squash to get spaghetti-like strands.
4. Place 2 cups spaghetti squash in each of 2 greased and floured 8 inch pie pans.
5. Put all other ingredients into blender. Blend well.
6. Pour equally over the squash in each pan. Bake for 1 hour at 350 degrees.
7. A crust will form on the bottom.

Spaghetti Squash Bread

Ingredients:

1 1/4 cups flour
4 tbsp. sugar
1 tsp. baking soda
1/4 tsp. cinnamon
1/4 tsp. nutmeg
1/4 tsp. allspice
Dash salt
2 med. eggs
2 tbsp. oil
1/4 cup orange juice
2/3 cup spaghetti squash strands, cooked
2 tbsp. raisins

Directions:

1. Stir together well, flour, sugar, baking soda, spices and salt.
2. Set aside.
3. Beat together, eggs, oil and juice, gradually beat dry ingredients mixture into egg mixture. Stir in squash and raisins.
4. Pour batter into 9 x 5 inch non-stick loaf pan that has been sprayed with cooking spray.
5. Bake at 350 degrees for 40 minutes until golden brown.
6. Makes about 20 slices, 65 calories each.

Beef Spaghetti Squash Bake

Ingredients:

1 lb. ground beef
2 lbs. yellow and or zucchini
1 cup sliced mushrooms
2 cups soft bread crumbs
1 envelope spaghetti sauce mix
2 eggs, beaten
1 cup shredded Cheddar cheese

Directions:

1. Preheat oven to 350 degrees.
2. Ungreased 2 quart casserole.
3. Brown ground beef; drain off excess fat.
4. Add squash and mushrooms; continue cooking 3 or 4 minutes or until squash softens, stirring often.
5. Stir in crumbs and spaghetti sauce mix.
6. Spoon into 2 quart casserole; sprinkle with cheese.
7. Bake 30 to 40 minutes at 350 degrees.

Scalloped Spaghetti Squash

Ingredients:

1 spaghetti squash, cut in 1/2" pieces
1 1/2 cups milk
3 tbsp. flour
3 tbsp. butter
1 1/2 tsp. salt

Directions:

1. Make a white sauce of the last 4 ingredients. Place the squash in a buttered baking dish and cover with the white sauce. Bake 1 hour at 375 degrees. The last 15 minutes of baking, add a mixture of Hi Ho or Ritz crackers with 2 tbsps. onion flakes.

Spinach and Spaghetti Squash Quiche

Ingredients:

1/2 cup frozen chopped spinach , thawed, drained and squeezed dry
1/2 cup cooked, shredded spaghetti squash
1 beaten egg
3 egg whites
1 (12 fluid oz.) can evaporated milk
1 cup mozzarella cheese
Cooking spray
1/3 cup bread crumbs

Directions:

1. Preheat oven to 350 degrees F (175 degrees C).
2. Pierce squash several times with a fork, and place in a microwave-safe dish. Microwave on high for 10 minutes, turn over, and continue cooking 10 minutes more. Squash flesh should be very tender inside.
3. Set aside to cool.
4. Cut squash in half lengthwise and scoop out seeds.
5. Shred 1/2 cup of squash and place in a mixing bowl. Stir in egg, egg whites, evaporated milk, mozzarella cheese, and spinach until well combined.
6. Spray a 9 inch pie place or quiche dish with cooking spray. Spread bread crumbs in the bottom and around the sides to coat.
7. Pour egg mixture into prepared dish.
8. Bake quiche in the preheated oven for 45 minutes, or until a toothpick inserted in the center comes out clean.
9. Allow to cool for at least 10 minutes before cutting.

Spaghetti Squash with Asparagus

Ingredients:

1 spaghetti squash, halved lengthwise and seeded
1 tbsp. extra-virgin olive oil, or as needed
2 tbsps. coconut oil, or more as needed
1 bunch asparagus, trimmed
5 leaves fresh basil, chopped
1 cup multi-colored cherry tomatoes, halved
2 tbsps. pine nuts

Directions:

1. Preheat oven to 400 degrees F (200 degrees C).
2. Line a baking sheet with aluminum foil.
3. Coat the inside of spaghetti squash with olive oil and place, cut-side down, onto the prepared baking sheet.
4. Bake in the preheated oven until squash is tender and a fork can easily puncture the flesh, 30 to 40 minutes. Remove baking sheet from oven and cool squash until easily handled, about 15 minutes.
5. Heat coconut oil in a skillet over low heat; cook and stir asparagus until tender yet firm to the bite, about 5 minutes.
6. Shred the squash flesh using a fork to create long strands that resemble noodles.
7. Mix squash and basil into asparagus, adding more coconut oil if too dry; cook and stir for 1 minute. Remove skillet from heat and mix tomatoes and pine nuts into squash mixture.

About the Author

Laura Sommers is **The Recipe Lady!**

She is the #1 Best Selling Author of over 80 recipe books.

She is a loving wife and mother who lives on a small farm in Baltimore County, Maryland and has a passion for all things domestic especially when it comes to saving money. She has a profitable eBay business and is a couponing addict, avid blogger and YouTuber.

Follow her tips and tricks to learn how to make delicious meals on a budget, save money or to learn the latest life hack!

Visit her blog for even more great recipes and to learn which books are FREE for download each week:

http://the-recipe-lady.blogspot.com/

Visit her Amazon Author Page to see her latest books:

amazon.com/author/laurasommers

Laura Sommers is also an Extreme Couponer and Penny Hauler! If you would like to find out how to get things for **FREE** with coupons or how to get things for only a **PENNY**, then visit her couponing blog **Penny Items and Freebies**

http://penny-items-and-freebies.blogspot.com/

Other books by Laura Sommers

- **Fruit Smoothie Recipes**
- **Smoothie Recipes to Relieve Anxiety and Depression**
- **Totally Bare Green Smoothie Recipes (Raw and Vegan)**
- **Healthy Cold and Chilly Vegetarian Summer Soup Recipes**
- **Paleo Soup Recipes**
- **Super Slimming Vegan Soup Recipes**
- **Tofu Recipes**

May all of your meals be a banquet
with good friends and good food.

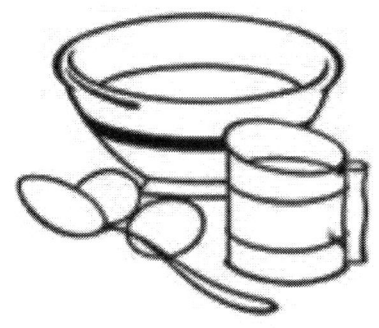

Printed in Great Britain
by Amazon